Crystals and Gemstones: Healing The Body Naturally

2nd Edition

By Crystal Muss

© **Copyright 2015 - All rights reserved.**

In no way is it legal to reproduce, duplicate, or transmit any part of this document in either electronic means or in printed format. Recording of this publication is strictly prohibited and any storage of this document is not allowed unless with written permission from the publisher. All rights reserved.

The information provided herein is stated to be truthful and consistent, in that any liability, in terms of inattention or otherwise, by any usage or abuse of any policies, processes, or directions contained within is the solitary and utter responsibility of the recipient reader. Under no circumstances will any legal responsibility or blame be held against the publisher for any reparation, damages, or monetary loss due to the information herein, either directly or indirectly.

Respective authors own all copyrights not held by the publisher.

Legal Notice:

This book is copyright protected. This is only for personal use. You cannot amend, distribute, sell, use, quote or paraphrase any part or the content within this book without the consent of the author or copyright owner. Legal action will be pursued if this is breached.

Disclaimer Notice:

Please note the information contained within this document is for educational and entertainment purposes only. Every attempt has been made to provide accurate, up to date and reliable complete information. No warranties of any kind are expressed or implied. Readers acknowledge that the author is not engaging in the rendering of legal, financial, medical or professional advice.

By reading this document, the reader agrees that under no circumstances are we responsible for any losses, direct or indirect, which are incurred as a result of the use of information contained within this document, including, but not limited to, —errors, omissions, or inaccuracies.

Contents

Introduction

Chapter 1 - Crystal and Gemstone Healing - Fact or Fiction?

    The Difference Between Crystal and Gemstone
    The New Age Science Behind Stone Healing
    Benefits of Crystal and Gemstone Healing

Chapter 2 - Most Common Health Problems That Crystals Can Heal

    Headache
    Mild Insomnia
    Heart Problems
    Blood Flow
    Stress and Fatigue
    Mental Troubles

Chapter 3 - Colors and Forms of Crystals and Gems

    The Psychology of Color
    Colors of Stones and Their Meanings
    Forms of Stones
        Rough Stones
        Polished
        Jewelry

Chapter 4 - Introduction to Chakra Points and Stone Healing

    What is Chakra?
    Chakra Points
    The Seven Color Chakra Layout and Popular Crystals for Chakra Balancing
    Popular Grounding Crystals

Chapter 5 - Step by Step Guide on How to Use Crystals and Gemstones to Heal the Body

Chapter 6 - Crystal and Gemstone Healing at Home

    How to Use Crystals
    Crystal Pendulum Dowsing
    How Does it Work?
    Good Advice Before You Begin

Getting Started

Chapter 7 - Feng Shui and Crystals

Rose Quartz
Clear Quartz
Jade
Hematite

Chapter 8 - Crystals and Meditation

Chapter 9 - Other Reminders When Using Crystals and Gemstones

Know Your Stones and Buy from Trusted Stores
Understand What They Do: Research, Research, Research
Crystal Healing is Not Meant to Replace Professional Healthcare
Your Private Crystal Database
  Name: Diamond

Conclusion

Introduction

Although medical science is always on the lookout for ways by which the improvement in health and cure of various diseases can be achieved, there's nothing wrong with finding other alternative ways to heal the body. People often choose these alternative ways because they are less invasive-- for example, medical procedures often involve insertion of intravenous fluids, administration of medications through injection, or worse, surgeries. These procedures are painful and costly, not to mention the risks included can cause permanent disabilities, or worst death.

A Brief History of Crystal and Gemstone Healing

The first recorded use of Crystals and Gemstone for healing dates back to the ancient times-- the pioneers are Ancient Sumerians and Egyptians. On top of using crystals and gemstones for health improvement and cure of ailments, they also believe that the use of the precious stones also bring protection from harm.

Back then, the use of crystals and gemstones are rooted on nothing but magic and superstition. A good example is when Egyptians used topaz to fight off night terrors. Greeks used amethyst to battle drunkenness and hangover, very fitting because the word amethyst means, "not drunken". In ancient China, jade was used to treat kidney diseases.

In this book...

Crystals and Gemstones have come a long way from when it was first used. This book aims for you to understand them more clearly and be able to guide you on the things you need to know when you use them to help improve your health and cure your body.

Come along on this fascinating and healing journey. You won't regret it.

Chapter 1 - Crystal and Gemstone Healing - Fact or Fiction?

You might find yourself asking this question: If Crystal and Gemstone Healing are just purely based on "Magic," why is it quickly becoming popular in health spas, and modern health clinics?

The fact is this: Although there is no Scientific Study confirming the benefits of Crystals and Gemstones, there is still science behind it.

The Difference Between Crystal and Gemstone

Crystal is a solid gem with a defined atomic structure. "Defined" meaning the atoms are arranged in an orderly, repeated manner. Crystals are symmetrical, so they come in twins.

Gemstones are made from minerals, and when they are polished, they can be used as jewelry. There are a lot of gemstones and each has a different interpretation (based on their colors) when it comes to healing.

The New Age Science Behind Stone Healing

Metaphysics teaches us the Crystals and Gemstones are "geometrically" perfect, from their exterior to their atomic structure. This perfect structure makes a gemstone and/or a crystal's Dominant Oscillatory Rate (DOR) very stable. But, what is DOR?

Dominant Oscillatory Rate dictates the body's balance. It is also referred to as vibrational frequency. And when there is balance, optimum health can be achieved. However, stresses, pollution, and illnesses can "mess" with our DOR. Further piece of knowledge is this: we are composed of varying DORs-- organs and cells have their own! It is safe to say that when stress and ailments come our way, our balance can be easily disrupted.

The good news is this: our body can easily attune with the correct vibrational frequency-- we just need to have a source. And crystals and gemstones, with their perfect and stable DOR, can be a very good source.

Furthermore, each crystals and gemstones have their own healing properties that can help a person with his or her specific condition. Precious stones are also believed to facilitate a life energy called qi. Qi is known as an invisible force that heals.

Benefits of Crystal and Gemstone Healing

Although the more complicated forms of stone healing employs specific properties (color, composition, etc.) and specific body parts, it is important to understand that ALL crystals and gemstones have one thing in common-- and this is their stable vibrational frequency. With this knowledge, you'll be able to incorporate Crystal and Gemstone Healing in your lifestyle just by having simple knowledge. And this simple knowledge will be discussed in this book in the future chapters.

The benefits of stone healing can range from something as simple as relieving short-burst of stress, to something as serious as liver diseases and endocrine imbalances. Other things that can be achieved through stone healing are occult-like opening the Third Eye, harmonizing the person's aura, and protection from spiritual attacks.

Chapter 2 - Most Common Health Problems That Crystals Can Heal

Crystal healing is one of the oldest forms of healing. It employs the use of crystals to balance the energy in the body and alleviate common ailments. Crystals are formed under high heat and pressure by atoms and molecules arranging themselves in a highly ordered and more definite lattice compared to other solid matter. Crystal healers believe that with their special internal composition, crystals have strong electromagnetic fields that can resonate throughout the body. They can store and transmit energy, and thus possess healing properties that can help one achieve harmony and balance with his/her physical, emotional, mental and spiritual health.

Different elemental crystals can bring different kinds of health benefits to the user, some of which we will talk about more in later chapters. To start with, here are the most common health problems that crystals can heal.

Headache

A headache may be caused by several factors. The good news is that many kinds of crystals can help you get rid of that dull ache. Try to find out the cause of your headache, whether they are a result of tension and stress, or a possible symptom of an underlying ailment. Headache, especially if coupled with stomachache, may also be caused by an internal imbalance in the body, between the Crown or Brow Chakra and Solar Plexus Chakra. You will learn more about chakras in the next chapter. Various types of crystals may aid in returning the body to its proper balance and alleviating the headache.

Mild Insomnia

For troubles with sleeping or constant restless nights in bed, try placing certain crystals under your pillow or somewhere near your bed. These can calm your nerves and even help you get rid of nightmares, allowing you a long and peaceful sleep.

Heart Problems

A large chunk of crystal healing is centered on improving the spiritual aspect of the person. As a person's spiritual health may affect the physical health, one of the causes of a person's ailment may be that their spiritual aspect is in turmoil.

Health problems concerning the heart, for example, may be attributed to a person's negative emotions or poor spiritual well being. Crystals that boost the Heart Chakra, like green or pink crystals, can help calm and bring about emotional balance. Color chakras will be discussed further in later chapters.

Blood Flow

Ailments that, in one way or another, concern the blood, such as painful premenstrual syndrome (also known as PMS), kidney problems and even other problems concerning the internal organs where blood flows through, can be eased by certain crystals. Many crystals are believed to be able to help remove toxins from the blood, improving the body's overall health. When trying to treat problems that concern one's internal physiology, healers would employ a specific healing layout (such as the Seven Color Chakra Layout) to place different-colored crystals on the different areas of a person's body. Take note that crystal healing is a non-invasive method.

Stress and Fatigue

On most days, many of us aren't really sick with a disease or ailment that needs medical treatment. Rather, the constant toils of life just keep us stressed and tired. At times like this, crystals can be a fast and easy way to obtain energy from the earth. Most people like to wear crystals around their necks not just for the said reasons, but also because they look pretty as accessory items as well.

Mental Troubles

Are you having trouble concentrating? Do you constantly feel like a scatterbrain with the way you easily forget things? Do you need to prepare your mind for a major study session? Some crystals can aid you in clearing your mind, organizing thoughts, and helping you focus. Some others may also improve your memory skills and concentration.

Chapter 3 - Colors and Forms of Crystals and Gems

The colors you see in a crystal are a result of a combination of atomic structure and the way the mineral interacts with the light. There are two basic types of color – ideochromatic, which are minerals like copper or chromium and allochromatic. Ideochromatic mineral colors are affected by the chemical composition whereas allochromatic mineral colors come from impurities, maybe only a few small atoms, of another element that is responsible for creating anomalies inside the crystal structure.

The colors that we see in opaque stones are from light frequencies that are not absorbed into the structure. On stones where the light is all absorbed, the stones appear black, whereas white stones fully reflect he color spectrum and will not absorb any light at all. If a crystal is translucent or transparent, the light rays that go into the structure are bent, refracted and slowed down by the way the atoms are arranged. Depending on how the atoms actually modify the light photons, the crystal may move an entire spectrum towards a slower frequency and will appear red or, if they shift towards a faster frequency, they will appear violet or blue.

With allochromatic stones, the small anomalies in the structure carry energy charges that pick up proton particles and form the coloration of the stone. When the color changes according the viewing angel, this is called Pleochromism and is created by the internal structures breaking up the light rays in different ways, depending on where the light goes into the crystal. Diffraction is the polarization of the light, where it changes speed and frequency and comes out of the crystal at all different angles.

The Psychology of Color

As humankind has evolved, so has the way our bodies react to light. Color therapy is one of the more important methods of holistic treatment these days and it is know that your personality is affected by different colors. This could be through conditioning or it could be through an experience with a color. Color vibrations also influence us, each one having its own rate of vibration, which correspond with the inner body vibrations. We also know that each part of the body resonates to different colors. Each color has psychological associations and can be linked to specific moods. Yellows, reds and oranges are warm colors, giving of energy, joy and excitement, where the blues, purples, and indigo colors are cooler and calmer, inducing a sense of relaxation. Below I will go into more details on the different colors and their meanings. To be able to perform correct stone healing you have to know the different forms and colors of crystals and gemstone. These features of stones can directly affect their healing properties.

Colors of Stones and Their Meanings

Red - Red is the color you'll have to choose if you want to improve your circulatory system. People who lack energy, confidence and the drive to pursue their dreams also gravitate towards this color because its flare is a symbol of stamina. Lastly, those who suffer from sexual dysfunction can also be helped by this stone color.

Indications of Red Energy Imbalances:

- Cold, congested or inactive conditions
- Difficulty moving, with circulation and with coordination

- Lack of energy, physically weak and exhausted

- Unable to experience life, either mentally or emotionally, as it should be, a real lack of enthusiasm or drive, lethargy and not comfortable with physical activity

- Feeling vulnerable or alienated, unable to maintain boundaries and drain easily when in company

Crystals that balance red energy are:

- Red Jasper
- Agate
- Snowflake Obsidian
- Hematite
- Black Onyx
- Black Tourmaline
- Bloodstone
- Pyrite
- Smokey Quartz

Orange - Orange is the color to be provided for sickly people who lack their appetite. Due to its vibrant aura, orange can stimulate food craving. Lastly orange is a good color to boost your creativity.

Indications of Orange Energy Imbalances:

- Physically rigid
- Restriction of feelings
- Disorders of the digestive system

- No focus
- No vitality
- Hanging on to memories, unable to step out of the past

Crystals that balance orange energy are:

- Red Jasper
- Camelian
- Amber
- Smokey Quartz
- Tigers Eye

Yellow - For people who are prone to feel depressed and those who always live in their busy schedules, the color yellow helps liven up the mood. It is also a very effective color to relieve a person from stress and burnout.

Indications of Yellow Energy Imbalances:

- Stress and stress related disorders such as indigestions, panic attacks, insomnia, muscle tension and headaches
- Nervous disorders
- Arthritis
- Food intolerances
- Allergic reactions
- Confusion, tension and worry

Crystals that balance yellow energy are:

- Yellow Jasper
- Citrine
- Golden Quartz
- Goldstone
- Pyrite
- Honey calcite

Green - The color of nature relieves tiredness of the eyes. It is also a good color for fertility. Those who are looking for balance can also turn to this color. This color is also associated with the heart.

Indications of Green Energy Imbalances:

- Invasive illness
- No control at any level
- Abnormal growths
- Claustrophobia or feelings of domination, feeling trapped or restricted
- A real need to be controlled or to be in control
- No self-discipline
- Confusion
- Isolation

Crystals to balance green energy are:

- Green Aventurine

- Rose Quartz
- Amazonite
- Aquamarine
- Emerald
- Fuschite
- Jade
- Lepidolite
- Mookite
- Peridot
- Rhodonite

Blue - For people who find it difficult to sleep, blue is the coolest color to incorporate in their stone healing. It is also good for people experiencing some sort of chaos in their life as the color has a very calming hue.

Indications of Blue or Indigo Energy Imbalances:

- Problems with the throat, such as laryngitis, sore throat or tonsillitis
- A block on inspiration and creativity
- Difficulty in communicating
- Becoming agitates

Crystals to balance blue or indigo energy are:

- Sodalite

- Blue Lace Agate
- Lapis lazuli
- Amazonite
- Apatite
- Kyanite
- Labradorite

Purple - When in need to use your imagination, the color purple can trigger its activity. It is also a good color for those who are depressed and those who lack energy.

Indications of Purple or Violet Energy Imbalances:

- A real need to sacrifice for other people, usually due to guilt or a sense of no worth
- Living in a world of illusion, fantasy or daydreaming
- Delusions and personal fanaticism, resulting in reality being reinterpreted
- Headaches
- Eye and ear problems
- Glandular imbalance
- No spiritual or mental focus
- Lack of concentration
- Unable to deal with change

Crystals to balance purple or violet energy are:

- Amethyst
- Fluorite
- Labradorite
- Lepidolite

Indigo - For those who seek to understand themselves better, it's advisable to use an indigo gem or crystal. This color is also good for developing intuition. See Blue above for indications of energy imbalances and stones to balance them out

Black - Although often times misunderstood as the color of death and evil, black for crystals and gemstones often mean mystery. If you want to be noticed, and yet do not want others to violate your space, black is the color for you. It is also the color of a person who maintains control, by not giving way any information to others. It indicates something that is lying dormant and is also connected to philosophical ideas and thoughts. Someone who continuously wears black may be trying to say that something is missing from his or her lives. Negative black believes that there is no longer anything to look for, that there is nothing there anymore but, at the real heart of it, black is the color of discipline. Discipline brings freedom, which can be extremely liberating. Black is associated with the root chakra, which is associated with the color red – See above for details of crystals to correct black energy imbalances.

White - White is a denser form of cosmic intelligence of brilliance. It has one fundamental quality – all colors are equal in white. White signifies supreme faith, fully derived from logic and reasoning and it conjures up feelings of hope. However, the downside is that the color white has one major enemy – itself. White jobs tend to be professions that are precise and streamlined, such as the banking industry, civil service and ergonomics.

Crystals to balance white energy are:

- Clear Quartz
- Selenite
- Golden Quartz
- Opalite
- White Howlite

REMINDER: Although colors do not really play any scientific value when it comes to healing, stone healers suggest that the "belief" of a person who seeks cure can set the mind, so that it'll work to gain an optimistic result.

Forms of Stones

When crystals are obtained from the earth and it was not processed in anyway, the crystal is said to be rough or unpolished. Mostly, rough gems and crystals are used as ornaments in a certain area to bring about positive vibe in the place. Since crystal healing requires that the stone directly touch your skin, you might want to purchase different polished stones, depending on your need and desire.

The most common form of polished stone used in crystal and gemstone healing are polished point (such as clear quartz) and tumble stones, which are tiny, very suitable to be placed on different parts of the body.

Rough Stones

These are natural stones, unworked and he same as they were when they came out of the rock they were living in. The surface of rough stone is irregular and contains a large amount of healing power. Rough stones can be gently placed on the body to focus the healing energies.

Polished

Polished stones have been tumbled, using a mixture of sand and water, to give them a smooth and rounded surface. Polished stones are used as touch stones and can be carried in a pocket. Because of their smoothness, they are used for gemstone healing as they can be put on the body, rubbed or held.

Jewelry

Jewelry that has been made from healing stones and crystals contains stones that are needed for energy. The design is important and the power of the stones is enhanced by the colors and the precious metals used. Gemstone jewelry can be created to provide vibrations for harmony, for specific health needs and to help you to maintain positive intentions for a number of blessings, including love, prosperity, protections and clarity.

A very good example of gemstone jewelry is birthstones. The origins of the birthstone go back to Egyptian times when each month was given a different gemstone or crystal. These also provide support for the astrological signs of the zodiac.

Chapter 4 - Introduction to Chakra Points and Stone Healing

It's been briefly tackled that for stone healing to occur, there must be a direct contact between the skin and the crystals and gemstones. Now, the question is where to place the stones so that you'll have the desired healing effect?

To answer that question, we must first discuss chakra and chakra points.

What is Chakra?

Chakra is a Sanskrit term that means "wheel". Psychics who can see them describe chakra as wheels of energy travelling in the body. Chakra too, are working in balance, if for an instance they are thrown out of their harmony, or if they were blocked, a person may feel restless and it may convert to physical manifestations of illnesses.

The imbalances and blockage of our chakra can be remedied by the perfect DOR of the crystals and gemstones.

Chakra Points

There are very many crystals that you can purchase from

traditional healing stores and jewelry stores. Even many online stores cater specifically to crystal and gemstone enthusiasts. For someone new to crystal healing, the wide selection may overwhelm you. A good way to start, however, is to choose from popular crystals and gemstones that are well received due to their price, availability and many healing benefits.

While most crystals hold many healing properties, they could be more effective in one specific area than others. Therefore, when looking for a crystal, it's best to at least have some idea on what kind of healing benefits you wish to obtain. A good way to start is to follow the Seven Color Chakra Layout, one of the most popularly followed healing grids, and to have at least one crystal for each color chakra.

The body has seven major chakra points, in this section we will discuss what will happen should those chakra points be imbalanced or blocked. We will also discuss their location in the body.

The Seven Color Chakra Layout and Popular Crystals for Chakra Balancing

Crystal deeply concerns the goal of energizing and cleansing the spirit. It relies heavily on the person's chakra system. The human body has seven major chakras or energy points, each corresponding to a particular color and a particular part of the body. These energy points can be hindered or disrupted, however, if a person is stressed, troubled or emotionally unstable. Disruption of chakras and energy points, in turn, can lead to physical ailments such as those listed in the previous chapter.

Crystal healing aims to cleanse and balance the chakras in order to alleviate emotional troubles, which will, in turn, ease physical ailments. By following the Seven Color Chakra Layout, a person may place crystals of the corresponding chakra color onto the appropriate areas of their body.

The First Chakra or the Root - The first chakra point is called "root". It can be found at the base of the spine, and in front of the tailbone.

The Base or Root Chakra is the first chakra of the system. It corresponds to the very base of the spine. This red chakra concerns the grounding and self-preservation of an individual. If you are a daydreamer, constantly having trouble concentrating, and dwelling more on things other than the present matter, then you may need to revitalize your first chakra in order to "bring you back to earth"; that is, to stabilize your overall self to keep you grounded and focused.

Anatomically, the Base Chakra controls the spinal column, adrenal glands, kidneys, colon and the nervous system. Lower body problems, constipation, osteoarthritis and obesity are physical telltale signs of poor Root Chakra.

Popular red chakra crystals and stones include the red calcite, which is also a good energizer; the red jasper, which can also help you through difficult situations, and the garnet stone that can stimulate your sex and love life.

When imbalanced or blocked: It can make a person feel fearful and anxious. This point is also associated with knee problems (including the hip and legs), obesity and sexual organs.

Colors of stones to be used: Red and Black

The Second Chakra or the Belly/ Sacral - Is found two inches just down the navel.

The Sacral, Navel or Spleen Chakra corresponds to the area around two inches below the navel, above the pubic bone. This orange chakra concerns creativity, passion, emotions and sexuality. Improving the Sacral Chakra may soothe negative emotions such as anger, fear, and guilt.

Anatomically, the Sacral Chakra controls the sexual organs of a person (including the mammary glands of women) and the organs nearby. A poor Sacral Chakra may lead to impotence, poor libido, muscle cramps, constipation, bladder, kidney and uterine ailments.

Popular orange chakra crystals include the amber, a fossilized tree resin that can strongly absorb negative energy, and the carnelian, which you can also place near your door to protect your home.

When imbalanced or blocked: A person may experience kidney problems, constipation, spasms of the muscles, and lower back pain.

Color of stones to be used: Orange

The Third Chakra or the Solar Plexus - It can be found two inches below your breastbone.

The Solar Plexus Chakra corresponds to the area below the chest, between the navel and the base of the rib cage. This yellow chakra concerns self-identity, confidence, humor, and warmth. If you constantly overwork yourself and have trouble finding self-fulfillment, then energizing your third chakra may help induce a more positive outlook.

Anatomically, the Solar Plexus Chakra controls the digestive organs – the stomach, pancreas, liver, gallbladder and even the diaphragm. As such, digestive problems like stomach ulcers, as well as allergies and diabetes, may indicate a poor Solar Plexus Chakra.

Popular yellow chakra crystals and gemstones include citrine, which is also a pendant well-used by merchants as it is believed to bring in cash; the tiger's eye, a stone of protection, and the golden topaz, a tension reliever and aura cleanser.

When imbalanced or blocked: A person may have problems with

his or her gall bladder, stomach, pancreas, small intestine and liver.

Color of stones to be used: Yellow

The Fourth Chakra or the Heart - Can be found at the very center of your chest and lightly above the heart.

The Heart Chakra corresponds to the center of the chest. This green or pink chakra concerns compassion, humanitarianism, love and forgiveness. A person with balanced Heart Chakra is affectionate, easy to forgive, and cares for worldly issues such as hunger and poverty.

Anatomically, the Heart Chakra controls the heart, lungs, thymus gland, lymph glands, blood circulation and the immune system. A poor Heart Chakra consequentially causes lung and heart ailments, asthma, and hypertension.

Popular green and pink chakra crystals include the emerald, which can promote intimate relationships; the green jade or nephrite, which can also be worn for protection and emotional balance, and the rose quartz, also known as the Love Stone as it brings about love and forgiveness to a person.

When imbalanced or blocked: A person with troubled 4th chakra point can experience heart symptoms like stroke, high blood pressure and difficulty in breathing.

Color of stones to be used: Green

The Fifth Chakra or the Throat - This chakra point is located at the depressed area of the collarbone, which is shaped letter "V".

The Throat Chakra corresponds to the throat area, near the bottom of the neck. This light blue or turquoise chakra concerns one's communication and self-expression. When this certain energy point is balanced, a person is artistic, contented, sociable and able to express himself/herself properly.

Anatomically, the Throat Chakra controls the esophagus, throat, thyroid gland, neck, mouth and teeth. Colds, stiff neck, throat problems, as well as hearing and voice problems may indicate an imbalance of the Throat Chakra.

Popular crystals for this chakra include the turquoise, which can also help protect you against outside negative forces such as pollutants, and the aquamarine, which is also a good supplier of strength and courage.

When imbalanced or blocked: It can cause ear infection, hyperthyroidism, sore throat, back pain and skin irritation.

Color of stones to be used: Blue

The Sixth Chakra or the Third Eye - Located on the forehead, in the area between the eyes.

The Brow Chakra or the Third Eye Center corresponds to the area between the eyebrows, at the third eye. This dark blue or indigo chakra concerns one's psychic abilities and mental capacity, such as knowledge, intuition, and concentration.

Anatomically, the Brow Chakra controls the brain, eyes, ears, nose, pineal and pituitary glands. Disrupted Brow Chakra may cause one to experience headaches, poor vision and hearing, hallucinations, nightmares and other mental problems.

Popular crystal for this energy point include the lapis lazuli, which can also be placed at the Throat Chakra; the amethyst, which can also be placed at the Crown Chakra, and the quartz, also known as the Master Healing Crystal because as a clear crystal, it contains all of the colors of the spectrum, and thus, can be used for every Chakra and to harmonize the overall balance of the healing layout.

When imbalanced or blocked: When troubled, a person can experience eyestrain, blurred vision, headaches, and worst, blindness.

Colors of stones to be used: Indigo

The Seventh Chakra or the Crown - Found at the very top of our head.

The Crown Chakra corresponds to the crown or the top of the head. This violet chakra concerns the cosmic energy of a person. It is the bridge between our physical and spiritual selves, and it affects our thought patterns, imagination and inspiration as well.

Anatomically, the Crown Chakra controls the brain, nervous system, and pineal and pituitary glands. Disrupted Crown Chakra may lead one to experience headache, confusion, depression, overthinking, and stress.

Popular crystals and gemstones for the Crown Chakra include the opalite, a milky stone that can open one's psychic abilities, and ruby in zoisite, which can also improve individuality and eradicate laziness.

When imbalanced or blocked: It can cause migraine depression and headache.

Color of stones to be used: White and purple

Popular Grounding Crystals
When performing the Seven Color Chakra Layout, having a grounding crystal is also useful to help stabilize yourself afterwards. Popular grounding crystals include tourmaline, which will also protect you from negative energies, and bloodstone, a red and green jasper that can help the mind focus.

Chapter 5 - Step by Step Guide on How to Use Crystals and Gemstones to Heal the Body

Now that you know about the different stone colors and what they signify, and you know the manifestations that can happen when different chakra points are blocked or imbalanced, it's time to learn about the step-by-step guide on stone healing.

Step 1 - Choose the Correct Stone

Depending on what you want to achieve, look up for the meaning of the color. Or if you already have physical symptoms, find out what chakra is being blocked and see what stone color you should use. Remember that you have to use polished stones, preferably tumble stones.

Step 2 - Clearing

As soon as purchasing the stones, make sure that you'll clear them. This is done so that you'll be certain there isn't negative energy that's lingering. The simplest way to clear gems and crystals is just to wash them with detergent and then rinsing them with running water, but you can also try the following:

Moonlight - Just leave the stone overnight where the moonlight can shine over it. Experts suggest that new moon and full moon are the best phase to clear stones. Just be careful-- don't leave the stones to the point that the sun has already shone. Sunlight tends to fade the colors of the stones and sometimes they even leave cracks.

Smudging - While cedar or sage is burning, let the smoke pass all around the crystal. Do this a couple of times to ensure that the stone is clear.

Burying - Bury your stones in a cup of dried herbs overnight. You can also bury them in the ground, especially if you feel like deep cleansing is needed.

Cleansing is performed whenever a crystal or gem is newly purchased, or when you think that having them does not make you feel good anymore. The duration and frequency can actually be a personal choice.

Step 3 - Programming

Programming or sometimes referred to as "dedicating" is a ritual done to maximize the stone's potential. All you need to do here it to make certain that the crystal or gem will do what you desire them to do.

The process is simple, you just have to hold the stones in your hand and feel its energy. And then think about your goal for the healing. Experts do it by closing their eyes and chanting a mantra; you can also perform it and make your goals your mantra. Do this step until you feel like the stone has already been programmed.

Step 4 - Laying of Stones

The healer does the laying of stones. He or she will ask you to lie down and then he'll start placing gems on your various chakra points. Even though you're only feeling one physical manifestation, the healer will still place various stones on all the chakra points to promote holistic improvement.

Chapter 6 - Crystal and Gemstone Healing at Home

For those who want to heal at the comfort of their homes, follow the first three steps in the previous chapter and replace step 4 with any of these methods:

Wear it close to the body - Turn your stone into an accessory or jewelry and place it as close to the chakra points as possible.

Use it while bathing - Place the gems or crystals in the water you will use for bathing.

Keeping it under the pillow - For those who have panic and anxiety attack, or those having insomnia, this method is advisable.

For those who have no physical problems, placing gemstones and crystals as ornament in the office or at home is known to drive negative energy and encourage the presence of the positive vibe.

And if you're seeking to improve your inner self, these stones can also be used in meditation.

How to Use Crystals

There are a number of ways that you can use crystals and gemstones and it is all down to personal preference as to how you use them. Some of the more popular ways are:

Worn as jewelry on the body or close to the body

Wearing them is the most common way of using crystals and gemstones and, even if you have no knowledge of their powers, you will often select jewelry that contains stones with a positive effect. While you should choose stones that suit your purpose, you should also listen to your intuition.

Crystals that are worn on or close to your body are used for protection or healing and tend to have an effect over the whole body and the energy field. It is not important where the stone is located in many cases, although placing it near to the area related to the purpose of the treatment will often result in it working faster and being more focused. The healing energies of the stone or crystal will always go where they are needed but you can direct the energy focus yourself, by placing it in a pocket or on a necklace or ring near where it needs to be.

The strongest effects of the stones will be controlled by the length of the pendant chain. One that rests at the base of the throat will have more effect things like creativity, communication and anything else that relates to the throat chakra but it will still give energy to the whole body and aura. A stone on a longer chain will affect the areas governed by a different chakra. There are those who believe that a crystal or gemstone worn on the right will provide influence over outside matters while those on the left are to do with receiving energy.

Laid under a pillow

There are a number of advantages to keeping a crystal under the pillow while you sleep, not least that certain crystals will help to combat insomnia. They can also help to ward off psychic attacks and nightmares while other crystals can help you to remember your dreams of help with astral travel or out of body experiences.

In the bath

Crystals can be placed either in the bathwater or around the edge of the bath and is a highly enjoyable method of using crystals. Bathing is a cleansing act, not just physically but on all four levels. It can help to wash the stresses of the day away, remove negative tensions and emotions. It can refresh, soothe and revitalize you as well as energizing you. If you put crystals in the bath, they will absorb negativity and the healing energy will go where it is needed and where it is directed. The best crystals to use are Clear Quartz, Rose Quartz and amethyst.

In meditation

The way a crystal is structured imparts order to the subtle body, which helps to quiet down and relax the mind. A problem is an issue that needs to be resolved and, by changing the way your thought processes work, the way that you think, you can sometimes come up with the solution to a problem that has been bothering you. You can either place them in front of you or hold them in your hands.

Placed strategically around the office or the home

Crystals can change the energy of a room or space, bringing the atmosphere to life and getting rid of negative energies. They can also bring harmony. You can put your crystals wherever you want, just use your intuition as to where you think they should be. Crystal clusters and raw crystals are better than the smaller single crystal at retaining the integrity of their energy and, because of this, they can hold on to more energy that is negative before they have to be cleansed.

Used to counteract pollution in the environment

Every single day we are faced with an onslaught of environmental pollution, causing our bodies harm. Plastics, radio waves, electricity and microwaves can all be harmful and they overload our bodies with stress. This makes us more likely to contract disease or illnesses. The geomagnetic field around the earth gives off a natural energy and this is being shielded by all these harmful substances, the ambient earth energy is slowly disappearing beneath a thick layer of pollutions. Added to the electrical devices that we have in our hands, we are becoming entrained, which means that our energy fields are down and we are more susceptible to illness or to becoming run down. Crystals can help to amplify our energy fields to help counteract the effects of pollutions and crystals are gaining in popularity in office structures where we are surrounded by computers, artificial lighting, metal, nylon and air conditioning, all of which give off harmful pollutants.

Making essences from gems

This is a liquid form of the energy patterns within a crystal and are made using water. Water has unique properties that make gem essences highly effective. In addition, because it is a liquid, it can be used in ways that solid crystals cannot. You must take care when making gem essences because some crystals and gemstones are toxic. If you are not sure, stick to Quartz crystals. You can make both gem water and gem essences. The water is made by putting a crystal into a bowl of water – spring water is best – and left for 10 hours or so overnight. As it is not as potent as gem essence, it can be safely drunk or sipped throughout the day. It can also be used in a bath, breathed in or sprayed on the body, in the home or on pets.

Gem essences are a little different and require the energy from the sunlight to activate. Put the crystal into a bowl and pour in just enough spring water to cover it. Put the bowl in the sun for about 2 hours and then half fill a small bottle with brandy – this is a preservative – and pour the gem water into the other half of the bottle. This is the "mother essence". If you want to make it idea for regular use, you should make a stock bottle, which is 50% brandy and 50% plain water. Add a couple of drops of the mother essence to the stock bottle and it can then be sipped, added to the bath, inhaled, or sprayed.

Crystal Pendulum Dowsing

How Does it Work?

A pendulum is nothing more than a tool that verifies what you subconscious already knows. It is an extension of our inner sense and it creates a visual representation of the way our inner energy changes. The pendulum works by amplifying tiny movements in the muscles in the energy that flows through our bodies. We are making the pendulum move on a subconscious level, not y obvious movements. Instead, it is miniscule reflex movement that we cannot see with the naked eye.

Good Advice Before You Begin

We should never, ever, underestimate the power that the human mind has. In order for pendulum dowsing to be effective, you must stay relaxed and your state of mind must be neutral. Let's assume that you are looking for the answer to a question and have asked your pendulum. There is always an emotional investment, at some level, in the answer you want ad the answer you receive. You may not get the answer that you want to get from the pendulum and, rather than tossing it to one side in disgust, stop and think. This your conscious mind affecting the answer, not the subconscious so you need to relax, clear your mind and start again – let your subconscious do the talking.

Examples of how you might use a pendulum:

- Asking a simple question that requires a Yes, a No or a Not Sure answer

- Pendulum dowsing with maps and lists

- Trying to locate chakras and balance them by pendulum dowsing over the body

Getting Started

First, you must choose a pendulum that feels right. This is vital because you will be working with it on a very close level and, as such, your connection has to be the same as any other type of relationship.

Hold your pendulum gently, between your forefinger and thumb. You must hold it lightly because tension will affect the results you receive – your conscious will be doing the work for you.

Now you must determine how your pendulum is going to respond to specific answers – N, Yes, Not Sure, for example. This is something akin to a control test so you need to ask your pendulum a question to which you already know what the answer is. For example, let's say your birthday is on January 1, so ask your pendulum "is my birthday on January 1?" You know that the answer to that question is yes so you need to monitor how the pendulum responds. Does it move in a clockwise circle, anticlockwise? Back and forth? That movement is the Yes answer. Now ask a question to which you know the answer is going to be No. You should be able to determine a very fine difference between this response and the Yes. This may not happen straightaway - a bit of practice may be needed first. Make sure that you are fully relaxed, have a neutral state of mind and are not concentrating too hard!

Effective answers are only as good as the questions that are asked and the technique used. If you ask a question that is vague, expect an answer that is not specific or definite.

Chapter 7 - Feng Shui and Crystals

Feng shui is an ancient Chinese philosophy of aligning the energy forms in our surroundings to harmonize all aspects of our lives – health, money, relationships, career, and so on. By orienting our physical lives the right way, we may influence the Universal Life Force to affect us positively.

Much of feng shui is about building your home and orienting furniture inside it in certain ways that will promote the entering and residing of good energy, as well as protection and defense against negative energy.

Crystals can also play a part in feng shui. By placing certain crystals in certain rooms or in your office, you may be able to bring in the positive energy of the Universal Life Force to help steer you and your family's lives in the right direction. Another plus is that crystals can be beautiful decorative pieces that bring color and texture into your home interior.

Feng shui can be difficult to learn, as there are many factors to consider when arranging objects, such as the elemental properties, colors, and bagua areas. The bagua is a commonly used feng shui diagram that identifies the energies in the different areas of your homes, each area thus corresponding to a specific aspect of your life.

Just like crystal healing for the body, the primary goal in feng shui with crystals is to bring balance among the energies in order to positively influence every aspect of your life. Listed below are popular, easy ways to orient crystals in your home.

Rose Quartz

Rose quartz is definitely a popular choice when it comes to feng shui. As mentioned in the previous chapter, rose quartz is also known as the Love Stone. Using rose quartz to adorn your home can help improve love within the family, as well as your relationship with others.

The best place to place a rose quartz is in the Southwest Area of your home, which is identified as the Love and Marriage Area by the bagua. You can also place a bowl of rose quartz crystals at the center of your home, or in your bedroom to ease you to sleep.

Clear Quartz

The clearer, the better. Just like its appearance, the clear quartz crystal is useful in cleansing and purifying the energy in whatever area it is placed. As such, you can place it almost anywhere you feel that may need some earth elemental guidance and clearing. Keep your quartz crystal shiny and clean.

Jade

Yet another purifying stone is the jade stone. It is a very popular stone that is widely sold in many different forms, from lucky charms to jewelry. In feng shui, jade is popularly used in carved figurines. Jade is also a stone that protects and brings the energies into harmony. As a stone belonging to the earth element, you can place a jade stone in any area of the home, except for the North and South bagua areas.

Hematite

Just by looking at its distinct appearance, you'd know already that the hard, heavy, shiny black hematite is not a mineral you'd want to mess with. In feng shui, hematite brings grounding and protection to a home. It balances surrounding energies, helping you to be calmer and more focused.

Placing hematite in the West bagua area of your home, which is the Children and Creativity Area, will help the children in your home pay more attention and concentrate better. You can also place the hematite in their rooms.

For a more stable career and life overall, decorate the North bagua area of your home, also known as the Life and Career Path Area, with hematite. You can also place some in your office, as well.

To utilize the protective power of the hematite, place some tumbled rock hematites near your front door, either inside or outside.

Chapter 8 - Crystals and Meditation

What usually accompanies the Seven Color Chakra Layout is a session of meditation. While you place the appropriate crystals on each of the chakra areas of your body, clearing your mind and basking in the silence will facilitate better energy transmission of your crystals.

Meditation holds many great benefits to a person. Physically, it helps you relieve stress and tension within your body. Spiritually, you become calmer and more enlightened. Emotionally, you are given a chance to forget and let go of negative emotions. And mentally, you clear your mind temporarily from noisy thoughts and troubles. Overall, you reach into your deepest soul and try to find your inner being.

Different people may find different ways of meditation that work for them. The primary elements to keep, however, are silence, a relaxed physical body, and a clear, calm mind. You can perform breathing techniques, chant words or sounds, do yoga, and even visualize calm sceneries, situations or abstract things like the flow of crystal energies into your being.

Crystals can be incorporated with meditation either by placing them on your body, especially on the Heart Chakra and Third Eye

Chakra; holding onto them with your hand and feeling their energy transmit through you; wearing them as a charm or jewelry, or having them placed near you as a point of focus.

Chapter 9 - Other Reminders When Using Crystals and Gemstones

Now that you have learned so many things about crystal healing, here are some general guidelines to remember.

Know Your Stones and Buy from Trusted Stores

With so many varieties of crystals and stones in the market, you may find it hard to identify them right off the bat. Therefore, it is encouraged to read about the different crystals. Start with the popular ones or the ones you are interested to have. You can find many books and online articles about crystals and gemstones.

Having as much knowledge as you can gather will help you especially in your purchasing. Buy from trusted stores that introduce their crystals for what they are. Some crystal sellers may try to fool you into buying their fake products. For example, citrine is a rare crystal that can be hard to find, as most that are sold in the market are actually heat-treated amethysts. Don't be afraid to prod and question crystal merchants until you believe that their products are 100% genuine. After all, you only want to get your money's worth.

Understand What They Do: Research, Research, Research

It is important to differentiate crystals and stones from one another. Before you use anything for your healing grid or feng shui, read up or consult with an expert on the nature of the crystal, its physical properties and its healing properties. Randomly using crystals may sound harmless, but remember: some crystals can be toxic. You'll have to be careful especially when making crystal water, infusing crystals with massage oils, and cutting open or engraving crystals.

Crystal Healing is Not Meant to Replace Professional Healthcare

Although crystals have healing properties, by now you should have learned that most of crystal healing relies on treating the soul and balancing the energies within your body. Crystal healing is not meant to replace the scientifically based healthcare of licensed specialists. Crystals are not meant to replace medicines and drugs.

Your Private Crystal Database

At this point, I would like to provide a database for you to use as a quick reference for some of the crystals and the stones that you'll encounter on you journeys into New Age or Rock Shops across the world. It can be daunting and intimidating to be in a place with so many options without knowing what it is you're truly looking for out of the stone. You'll find them anywhere you go and you'll get a brief history and look at the stone. When it comes to crystals, there are numerous possibilities for you to acquire, but you're bound to find something that is going to work for you. Remember also that there are more stones out there than have been compiled on this list for you. Be sure to always be searching for the stones that are going to help you with what it is you're searching for out of life and not just because they're pretty.

Name: **Amethyst**

Variations: Amethyst is uniquely purple and is one of the dominant purple gemstones in the world.

History: Used heavily by the ancient Egyptians, it was a popular stone in antiquity and really made an impression on the Greeks who though it would keep intoxication away from them if they drank with an amethyst in their cup.

Qualities: Amethysts are renowned for working with head pain and any kind of mental issue. Blood sugar, brain imbalances, encouraging healing, and psychic stimulation are all qualities that you can expect to find with Amethyst.

Chakra Work: Stimulates the third eye Chakra that really opens you up during meditation for spiritual and mental insight.

Name: **Agate**

Variations: Numerous variations, in practically every color you can think of

History: Agate has been a popular stone for humanity since the dawn of time. You can find the fingerprints of agate in the jewelry, artwork, and decorations of humanity all across the globe and it carries with it that allure and that value to the current era.

Qualities: Depending on what kind of Agate you get, you can really work with it in any way and it will retain multiple qualities for you when you're going on a walk. When you're in a rock shop or at new age store, have a chat with the owners if they're into crystal work and ask them what agate they would suggest for you. They'll be more than willing to explain the difference. There are just too many to go into detail with here.

Chakra Work: Depending upon the color of the Agate you acquire, you can work with any of your Chakras. It all depends upon what it is you're looking to accomplish.

Name: **Amazonite**

Variations: Amazonite is exclusively green.

History: Although it takes its name from the famous Amazon River, the stone amazonite is almost exclusively mined in Russia. It has been found in Colorado, but it is really a rare stone and it has been popular ever since its discovery. It has been a round for a long time and is as beautiful as it is timeless.

Qualities: A stone for inspiration, you can carry this stone around with you and you'll be gin to notice that you're starting to have stronger will power and that you're ability to communicate is increasing.

Chakra Work: When it comes to your Chakra work, you should really associate this stone with your Heart chakra. This is going to help with healing, balance, serenity, and tranquility in your life.

Name: **Aquamarine**

Variations: Aquamarine is actually a blue variation of beryl, so you'll only find cyan.

History: This beautiful and lovely stone has actually had a very long and celebrated presence in the history of the world. It has been found in most areas that are prime mining locations and have spread across the world, adorning jewelry and decorations everywhere they land.

Qualities: As the name might imply, it's all about fluids. It helps you retain fluids in your body, ease your body if it's suffering from nerves or a cough. It's all about keeping you running regularly and successfully, mentally and physically.

Chakra Work: Since its most defining characteristic is the beautiful blue quality that the stone retains, it focuses on the Throat Chakra for most of your work. It helps you with communication and getting your ideas across, getting your presence to flow.

Name: **Bloodstone**

Variations: Bloodstone is actually a green stone with injections of red that give it the droplets of blood color. You can find some with yellow inclusions, which are called plasma.

History: Given the rather sinister name, bloodstone has been a part of history and dark rituals that involve the darker arts of magic. It has adorned rings and has been a warrior's stone for many cultures that revere the shedding of blood and the necessary acts of violence in life.

Qualities: This stone is all about the blood and everything that holds blood and pumps it. This stone wants your body working perfectly and it wants you to be at the best possible level that you could be. It's a blood cleaner and helps your blood circulation if you carry it with you.

Chakra Work: Given the dominant green color, this stone could be used with the heart chakra or the root chakra if you really want to draw out the red in the stone.

Name: **Carnelian**

Variations: Carnelian comes in a distinct reddish orange color

History: Carnelian is one of the oldest stones that we have record of and it's everything that you could possibly want in the ancient world. From the bold color to the striking presence it makes in jewelry, carnelian has been the rage ever since. Whether you were a high priest or you were a ruler, this was the beautiful stone you wanted.

Qualities: This is a stone that is used to keep you focused in the now, stimulating your curious side and pushing your attentions to keep you present in what you're actually doing and not wandering mentally. It also is great for your digestion if you keep it with you as you go about your business.

Chakra Work: This is an excellent stone for your root chakra, your sacral chakra, and your solar plexus chakra. All of these are greatly tied to carnelian and will help you when you're meditating and working on your chakras.

Name: Diamond

Variations: Clear or rose

History: What is there to say about diamonds that we don't already know. Since this beautifully clear crystal was hewn from the earth it has been the captivation and the wonder of every culture that has found them in their presence. It has predominantly been a stone that has come from Africa and has been heavily exploited.

Qualities: Diamonds work great for mental energy and are one of the healing stones that are employed heavily to remove toxins, poisons, and anything that might be wrong with your brain. By keeping a diamond on you, you're a very rich person, but you've also got a lot of healing flowing through you.

Chakra Work: Diamonds are mostly used for your crown chakra and to help you make contact with the greater cosmic awareness that is available to you. You can utilize it to really get to the root of some of your issues.

Name: **Emerald**

Variations: Green

History: Emeralds have been popping up all across the human civilization and has been quickly incorporated into the jewelry and the ceremonies of those that are in higher power and higher positions in society. The island of Ireland is known as the Emerald Isle, but that's due to the incredibly striking green color that the island has. There are no actual emeralds mined from Ireland.

Qualities: Emerald is a stone that is all about healing. It's great for helping your body open up and it's even better if you're looking to inspire loyalty and success in your love life. By keeping emerald on you, you're certain to have a better body and a better relationship with those around you.

Chakra Work: When it comes to emerald, the matters of the heart chakra are best inspired and dealt with if you're going to utilize emerald in your meditational practices.

Name: **Fluorite**

Variations: Due to imperfections, fluorite takes on the color of that is represented in the imperfection of the crystal. It is lovingly called the most colorful crystal in the world because it can take on any color that is represented in an impurity within the stone.

History: Fluorite has been a popular and quite confusing stone to our ancestors who were frequently baffled and confused by what it was that they were mining up from the earth. It has been known and confused with many different stones, but it has always had a presence in the history of our human civilization.

Qualities: Fluorite is commonly known as a crystal of the mind and is great when it comes to enhancing your memory, intelligence, wisdom, insight, and your focus. It's a stone that you want to carry with you if you're looking to be on the top of your mental game.

Chakra Work: It varies when it comes to fluorite because it has so many variations. You can really work with it in whatever way you need to. This makes it fluid and perhaps not the best stone for chakra work in general.

Name: **Garnet**

Variations: It varies from a dark purple to a bright red

History: No matter where you go in the world, garnets have been popular among the ruling class and the holy men of the local civilization. It's the kind of stone that has stuck out forever and is still drawing attention when it's formed into jewelry.

Qualities: This is a stone of great health and protection. For those that are into kundalini meditational practices, this is the stone for you. It builds up an internal fire and brings all of your creative and inspirational energy to life whenever you have it on you.

Chakra Work: This is a grounding stone that works very well with both your root chakra and your solar plexus chakra.

Name: **Hematite**

Variations: Silver or slightly red

History: The name for hematite comes from the Greeks who called it blood. It's the kind of stone that sticks around heavily utilized by the Greeks and all the cultures they inspired and grew to trade with across the world. You could find hematite as a cheaper stone for less expensive jewelry.

Qualities: This is a stone that serves to protect the person that carries it with them and is also greatly utilized to stimulate the health benefits of being fit and strong. It is also heavily utilized in the aura cleansing community and acts as a protector against negative energy that is around you.

Chakra Work: When it comes to chakra work, hematite isn't utilized as much as other stones, but it has a strong presence with your crown chakra.

Name: **Jade**

Variations: Jade is commonly green, but the hue can differ

History: Jade had played an enormous role in the cultures of Asia and has been one of the defining stones in their society and in their culture that has radically influenced their art, culture, and the way they design jewelry and other icons of beauty and influence.

Qualities: Jade is a stone of ambition, just as it was in ancient China and India, that quality rings true today. It's the kind of stone that you want around your neck and with you no matter where you go. It's a stone that is going to help you accomplish your objectives.

Chakra Work: Due to the power that this stone has to harness ambition and to turn it into a weapon for good, jade is commonly utilized for work that needs to be done with the heart chakra and the throat chakra.

Name: **Jasper**

Variations: Jasper can be found in a multitude of colors, mostly green, yellow, red, and brown.

History: There has been a lot of references to jasper through the history of the world and it has been very popular in cultures such as the Assyrians, the Hebrews, the Greeks, and the Romans. You can find a multitude of references and it has always been utilized as a craftsman stone, whether to make ornamental décor or jewelry for the owner.

Qualities: The qualities of jasper change depending upon which color you're utilizing for your presence or your meditation work, but all of them have their various qualities. You can use green to stimulate your connection with others, or red to ground you, or yellow to boost your energy and your presence in the lives of others. It all depends upon the stone that you're carrying with you.

Chakra Work: Once more, to sound like a broken record, it all depends upon the color you select. It can be utilized for root chakra, solar plexus chakra, or heart chakra, depending upon the color that you're using for your work. Decide which area you want to work with and then start using it.

Name: **Jet**

Variations: Jet is always black.

History: When it comes to jet, the culture that loved and adored jet the most was the Romans. They utilized it in every facet of life that they could get away with using it as. They made jewelry, cameos, and even used it in their use of magic. It has made a presence in many other cultures, but really came back to life in the Victorian Era when it was popular for jewelry.

Qualities: Jet is a stone that is used for those that are practitioners of the magical arts and are looking to be more attuned to the spiritual world. It will help you with your spiritual energy and keeping your body in tune with what it is you're looking to find. This stone is going to help keep you attached to the energy around you.

Chakra Work: Jet is not a stone that is commonly utilized in chakra work and is rarely brought in for meditational properties.

Name: **Lapis Lazuli**

Variations: Lapis Lazuli is a blue stone with flecks of yellow and gold within it.

History: Lapis Lazuli first makes an enormous appearance with the Egyptians who were struck with love and wonder for the stone. Whoever they encountered saw the beauty and power of the stone and incorporated it into their jewelry, art, and icons that were used in matters of state and in religious forums. Since the ages of antiquity, lapis lazuli has remained a stone of jewelry and art.

Qualities: This is a highly emotional stone that is going to help break through any blocks that you have. It's going to help you convey your emotions to others successfully and it's wonderful at eliminating negative energy and pushing away negative energy that might be plaguing you. It is also heavily utilized in healing and meditational uses.

Chakra Work: when you're looking to use lapis lazuli, those who are interested in maintaining their throat chakra and their third eye chakra mostly utilize it. This is a powerful stone that is often used in meditation practices.

Name: **Malachite**

Variations: Malachite is a distinctly green stone.

History: The tribal nations of the Holy Land and the Hittite Empire first took notice of this distinct stone that has been mined in Israel for ages. It has made its appearance for a very long time, working as a pigment and a stone that has been incorporated into jewelry for its distinct and unshakable color.

Qualities: This is a stone that is great at purging negative energy and opening up all the blocked emotion that might be lurking within you. It's going to give you greater insight into the events of your life and really open your eyes to the things around you that you might have been missing.

Chakra Work: This is a stone that is used for both the solar plexus chakra and for the heart chakra. It's a stone that is excellent to utilize when you're trying to get rid of blocks and open up your solar plexus.

Name: **Moonstone**

Variations: Moonstone is a stone that can take on the impurities of other stones around them, so it can take on multiple colors but always in faded and subdued colors that aren't as dominant as they might be.

History: The Romans admired moonstone and they believed that moonstones were made by the solidifying of moonlight and forcing it into a stone. It has been a representative for lunar deities since then and it has made an appearance in decorations and jewelry for many nations and has continued to endure in popularity to this day.

Qualities: Moonstone is most powerful when you couple it with lunar events and heavenly signs. It's the stone that is working heavily in your emotions and is all about developing your inner strength and cultivating a your psychic abilities. It's going to help you maintain some harmony throughout your day.

Chakra Work: When you're working with moonstone, you're probably going to utilize it the most when you're working on your crown chakra to keep you in tune with the cosmic order.

Name: **Onyx**

Variations: It's mostly black, but you can find red and yellow variations as well.

History: Onyx has been extremely popular for a long time because of its strange, enchanting darkness that has made cultures all across the world feel drawn to its power and presence. It's a stone that has popped up again and again in its multiple varieties in jewelry and decorations. The striking darkness of onyx has made it a favorite among artists.

Qualities: Onyx is going to really come into play on days that you're looking to really get some mental clarity and some objective thinking on matters. Its a decision stone that is going to help control your emotions and passions. It's going to also push away negative thinking and help you find the answers that you seek, no matter where it is you're searching. It's going to push away stress so that you can come to the conclusions that you need to.

Chakra Work: When you're working with onyx I would suggest that you utilize it best with the third eye chakra and really do some searching for it. Explore in the spiritual world with an objective and clear head. Get the answers you want.

Name: **Opal**

Variations: There are a lot of varieties when it comes to opal, ranging from dark to light and extremely colorful. It's usually always mixed

History: As early as 4,000 BC, Ethiopia has been working with Opal and it has made a presence in the ancient world ever since it was being mined from the earth. The way it diffracts light makes it exceptionally colorful and sparkle on a level that you don't find in natural, raw stones. It has made it stick out in jewelry and decorations alike for centuries.

Qualities: The great thing about opal is that you can find colors that work for multiple different reasons that you need. Whatever it is you're looking to inspire, opal will find a way to harness that in you. All of them regulate certain health benefits and it really comes down to what it is you need. Ask your local stone shop owner for an opal that will work for you.

Chakra Work: Just like the qualities and the colors of opal, you can use them for a wide variety of uses depending upon what it is you're looking to work with in your chakra and meditation work.

Name: **Peridot**

Variations: Peridot is always a distinct greenish yellow.

History: This ring's distinct green appearance has given it a special place in the presence of royalty and those that are interested in having something striking and gorgeous in their presence. You'll find this ring in many cultures as a fairly inexpensive work that was available for nobles and wealthy citizens.

Qualities: This is a ring of regeneration and of recovery. It's all about keeping the negative energy that comes from emotional, spiritual, or physical pain that might be plaguing your body. Carry this with you if you're looking to find some help with getting over the tension and troubles that are plaguing you.

Chakra Work: When it comes to Peridot, you're going to find that it works best with your heart chakra and really has the ability to open you up and get some serious work done when you're meditating. It's great at building up the energy you need.

Name: **Rhodonite**

Variations: Rhodonite is a mixture of rosy red to a bold pink.

History: Rhodonite is a stone that is very hard to ignore and it is very distinct when you see it. The bold pink that it commonly associates itself with has been the fixation of those looking to decorate or make affordable, yet striking jewelry and that's the presence that Rhodonite has made throughout history. You can find it in affordable jewelry and décor for those who have the money to spend on something truly beautiful.

Qualities: If you're looking to deal with a lot of mental dissonance and chaos, then Rhodonite is going to help you with just that. Whether you're looking to alleviate a certain amount of chaos that is causing unrest or just perpetrate a center of calm and confidence, you'll be able to. This stone is great at pulling away confusion an anxiety and help you see what it is you need to truly work on.

Chakra Work: Rhodonite is very popular for those looking to work with the third eye chakra, helping to push away any kind of mental confusions that might be clouding their pursuit of higher knowledge. It has also helped with the crown chakra. It all depends on which you need to utilize.

Name: **Quartz**

Variations: There are innumerable variations when it comes to quartz. Any color that you can imagine has a manifestation in quartz and that makes it an extremely versatile stone for anyone.

History: Quartz has been a massive influence in history and it has been one of the stones that has been used in so many art and jewelry projects that it's incredibly common for people to find and acquire. It's something that's full of possibilities when it comes to art and jewelry and the entire world is full of it. Whether it's ancient or modern, quartz is everywhere.

Qualities: Something that you're probably interested in when you're looking to quartz is mental stillness. There are a lot of different kinds of quartz that you can carry around with you, but they all have this same factor among them that they're excellent for cultivating a mental stillness if you carry it on you. So once more, depending upon what it is you need from your quartz, you can adjust the style and color and type, but they'll all give you that wonderful mental stillness.

Chakra Work: For those looking to utilize quartz in their chakra work, it's actually not that common due to the variations that are available. Again, you can specify what chakra you desire to work with and find a variation that will be suitable to the task, but other than that, they're all pretty low level stones.

Name: **Rhyolite**

Variations: Rhyolite is not a very lustrous or colorful, but it is very common and very useful.

History: Rhyolite was a vastly important to Native Americans who extensively quarried and picked up rhyolite so that they could use it for tools and instruments, even weapons of war. It was rarely used as jewelry, however it was a popular later on as a popular stone.

Qualities: One of the popular uses of rhyolite is that it reminds you of the value of yourself. It brings your emotions to an equivalent, but any form of question of self worth is brought to an end. It enhances your love and it brings your spiritual and your mental powers together as one.

Chakra Work: Rhyolite is super important for those working on their root chakra so that you can keep yourself together.

Name: **Ruby**

Variations: Ruby is a distinct, deep, blood red that is unmatched by any other stone out there. You know ruby when you see it.

History: The Kingdom of Macedonia was lucky enough to be the one nation in Europe that was predominantly gifted with the presence of rubies in their land. Because of that, they were given a huge amount of wealthy that generated from the mining, cutting, and polishing of rubies throughout history. Ruby has been the desired stone of men and women of power for generations who want to ensure that their strength is undoubtedly shown through their magnificent stone that's on their jewelry, rings, swords, and clothes.

Qualities: Rubies are commonly associated with the color that they portray in their bold appearance. They are given strength to those who carry them and they are also heavily influenced in the matters of romantic endeavors, helping you find and associate with desired people. You can also wear rubies if you have a blood deficiency to try and help circulation or cleaning of the blood. Those who wear rubies on their personages are often associated with wanting to draw power to them.

Chakra Work: Ruby has been strongly associated with the heart chakra and has been used for this specific purpose by most who work with it, regardless of the stone's color. Of course, you can always use it as a root chakra stone as well, but it's commonly associated with the heart chakra.

Name: **Sapphire**

Variations: Blue and pink both are extremely bold.

History: Sapphires are extremely popular among those who love the color blue and has been the best known as gemstone for jewelry. It's one of the best stones that has been utilized in jewelry. It's one of the great stones throughout history in every culture that could get them.

Qualities: By carrying around sapphire, you're going to be cultivating inner spiritual peace and a higher metabolic rate; this is going to do it for you. There are a lot of people who promote sapphires as a great stone for building up your psychic potential. Over all, it's aligned with spiritual enlightenment.

Chakra Work: Because of the remarkable blue quality of sapphire, there is a strong tie to the throat chakra when it comes to using sapphire in your meditational practices. Use this to really get energy flowing from you to the world and people around you.

Name: **Tourmaline**

Variations: Tourmaline has been distributed into so many different colors that are vivid, bold, and gorgeous. Whether you have the original pink or one of the many variations, it's beautiful. It comes in black, red, green, blue, and a unique color called watermelon, which is green on the outside and pink at the center.

History: Tourmaline has been found in its many varieties all across the world and it has been making an appearance in courtrooms, palaces, and anywhere rich and lavished for a very long time. It's one of the stones that has helped distinguish the rich and powerful from the poor and weak since it was first mined.

Qualities: Since there is a wide variety of tourmaline out there, you can bet that each one has a unique property that it helps and guides with. You're going to want to find one that helps what you're specifically looking for. There are so many unique colors and kinds that you're bound to find one that really helps you out. Plus, there's always the bonus that they're gorgeous.

Chakra Work: Do to the massive amount of varieties that tourmaline comes in, you can find one that works with practically every chakra that you have. It's a very versatile and powerful stone that you'll be harnessing the strength from in any meditation session.

Name: **Turquoise**

Variations: Turquoise is always a pale, milky blue that is distinctly classified as turquoise.

History: Turquoise has made a huge impact on the Native American cultures, but it's been around for an extremely long time all across the world. Its distinct color has made it hugely popular among jewelers and decorations all across the world. It's something that has been all around the world. You can find it from everywhere that makes in any way contact with the middle east where it has been discovered a long time.

Qualities: There is something about turquoise that has always made it a very protective and a very loving stone to the person who carries it. It wants to protect you from the environment, whether it's negative energy you fear or it's physical dangers. Turquoise is going to give you alertness and wisdom to find and avoid anything that might cause harm to you.

Chakra Work: When it comes to turquoise, this is a stone that is heavily utilized with the throat chakra to help regulate the flow of communication and energy to the world around you. Use this to open up your flow.

I strongly hope that this list of crystals that are fairly common for you to find in any store across the world will help you with the work you want to implement with crystals in your daily life. Remember that each has their own special prosperities and that there is plenty more to learn about when it comes to the fascinating and the magnificent world of crystals. Be aware that on your journeys you're likely to come across more stones and the different variations that are available for you to utilize. Go ahead and take advantage of the opportunity and learn all you can about them. They're a fascinating topic to study and they'll help you with all of your chakra work and your meditation practices. You're bound to find something here that is going to help you with exactly what you're looking for. Whether it is a specific chakra that you're looking to work with or you just need a stone to carry with you on your journeys, there's something here for everyone.

Conclusion

I hope the lessons presented in this book will be able to help you in your quest to heal your body using crystals and gemstones.

As a final note, please maintain a positive belief on the effects of the stones in healing the body, because the more optimistic your views are, the more positive effective they will have on you!

Good luck and happy healing!

You May Enjoy My Other Books!

TAROT: Fortune Telling and Mind Reading Secrets

hyperurl.co/tarot

MIND READING: Clairvoyance and Psychic Development

hyperurl.co/mindreading

Chakra For Lovers: Pleasure Guide Through Healing For Couples

hyperurl.co/chakralovers

RECOMMENDED READING

CRYSTAL HEALING ENERGY

smarturl.it/ccboxa

CHAKRA HEALING EXPOSED

smarturl.it/chakra

Tantric Sex and What Women Want - Box Set Collection: Couples Communication and Pleasure Guide

hyperurl.co/sexwomenwant

Liver and Gallbladder Detox: Natural Body Cleanse

hyperurl.co/liver

Made in the USA
Middletown, DE
04 December 2023

44582946R00040